# MEDICAL EXCELLENCE FOR A CHANGING COMMUNITY

# MEDICAL EXCELLENCE FOR A CHANGING COMMUNITY

## HOW CHICAGO'S SINAI HEALTH SYSTEM DEVELOPED AND ADAPTED

MAXWELL P. WESTERMAN, MD

MEDICAL EXCELLENCE FOR A CHANGING COMMUNITY

*How Chicago's Sinai Health System Developed and Adapted*

ISBN   978-1-5445-0380-6 *Paperback*
       978-1-5445-0381-3 *Ebook*

# CONTENTS

# FOREWORD

Sometimes, the hardest path is the most rewarding. Not in monetary terms necessarily, but in the currency that counts: deep professional and personal satisfaction of doing the right thing for a greater good. Just ask any of the four thousand committed caregivers at Sinai Health System, Chicago's largest healthcare system, serving the most vulnerable communities of low-income individuals. The patients and clients who Sinai has served for the past century often face the most daunting social and health issues imaginable: violent crime at a rate of 3.5 times that of the city, unemployment rates that are as high as seven times the city's rate, chronic disease such as diabetes that can be as high as three times the national average, and a depression rate more than twice that of the rest of the United States. Since 1919, Sinai Health System caregivers have been committed to "seeing our communities thrive in health," to use the vision statement of Sinai Urban

Health Institute (the research division of the system), whether welcoming and treating a refugee family at a first health visit in the United States, caring for a premature baby as small as thirteen ounces and sending that baby home at more than six pounds, or providing children in the community an after-school safe haven. So, when Max Westerman, MD, came to me with the idea that the Sinai story needed to be told, I knew he was right. In a country where many communities struggle without hope, or where health is elusive, Sinai Health System has become a beacon of light for the 1.5 million people in our service area. Dr. Westerman has seen it all through his forty-eight years as staff physician and renowned researcher. The community, patients, clients, caregivers, and board of directors at Sinai Health System owe Dr. Westerman a debt of gratitude for his commitment, vision, and tireless work on producing the history of a cornerstone of Chicago: Sinai Health System.

*Karen Teitelbaum*

KAREN TEITELBAUM, PRESIDENT AND CEO,
CHICAGO SINAI HEALTH SYSTEM

# DEDICATION

## MORRIS KURTZON

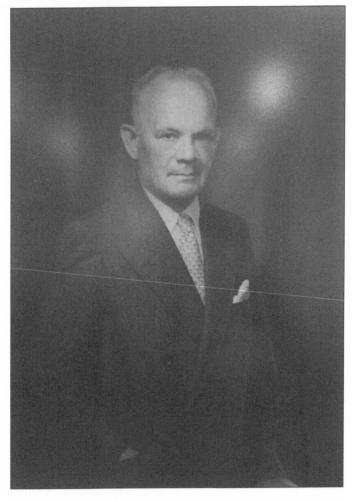

As the Founder of Mount Sinai Hospital, Morris Kurtzon deserves great credit for what Sinai is today. He never gave up against seemingly insurmountable difficulties and the greatest odds.

## STEVEN WHITMAN

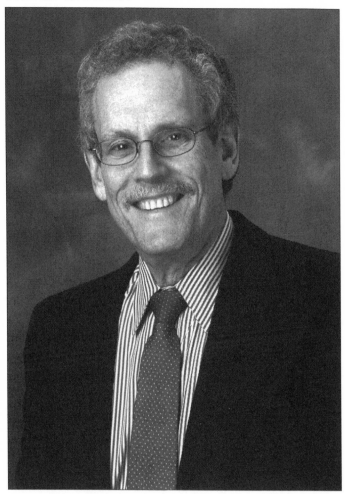

As the founder and director of the Sinai Urban Health Institute, Steven Whitman, besides being a truly fine individual, has made a major contribution to eliminate the health disparities that may occur in underserved communities.

# INTRODUCTION

The story of the Sinai Health System is the story of both a hospital and a health system which has provided healthcare to a local community for one hundred years. Since its inception, Sinai has provided healthcare for the North Lawndale community of Chicago, an underserved healthcare community. While doing so, Sinai has developed new and innovative ways to provide healthcare for such communities. Sinai Health System now serves residents in over one-quarter of Chicago.

SECTION ONE

# THE HISTORY OF SINAI HEALTH SYSTEM

*Chapter One*

___

# THE FIRST
# THIRTY YEARS

The first Jewish hospital in Chicago was Michael Reese, which was founded in 1865 by the first wave of German Jewish immigrants to the United States. The first attempt to found a Jewish hospital in North Lawndale, Chicago, was established in 1912. It was named Maimonides Hospital, after a twelfth century Jewish philosopher. The hospital became bankrupt after two years and closed in 1915. Four years later, Mount Sinai was founded, using the same building and organizational structure.

Mount Sinai Hospital was founded in 1919 by Morris Kurtzon as a response to the difficulties that the Jewish community had obtaining adequate healthcare. Between 1890 and 1914, over 200,000 Jews from Russia, Poland, and the Austro-Hungarian Empire fled to Chicago to escape religious persecution. They settled in North Lawndale, a section of Chicago that eventually became the largest Jewish settlement in Chicago.

While the first wave of Jewish immigrants, the German Jews, were now solidly middle class and well integrated into American society, the new wave of settlers was poorer and kept strong ties with their religious and ethnic backgrounds. There were no hospitals that supported their specific medical and religious needs.

## MORRIS KURTZON

Morris Kurtzon was the founder of Mount Sinai Hospital. Mr. Kurtzon was born in 1875 in Lithuania, immigrated to Chicago, and became a successful businessman. He first served as vice president of the platers' union for Chicago metalworkers before founding the Garden City Manufacturing Company in 1898.

Kurtzon's dream was to establish a hospital for the local community. The main goal of the hospital would be to provide adequate healthcare for the new Eastern European community of Jewish immigrants. He wanted a hospital to support the culture, language, and religious practices of these new immigrants. It was also meant to be a home for Jewish physicians.

In 1918, Kurtzon bought the bankrupt Maimonides grounds and buildings. Kurtzon devoted much of his time to planning and designing new facilities. He personally paid for most of the renovations.

The community contributed financially to the new hospital. The Jewish United Fund (JUF), an organization dedicated to serving the Jewish community, contributed significantly. The hospital also received funding from charitable groups, such as the Children's Aid Society of the Hospital, which was formed in 1918, prior to the hospital opening. In its inaugural year, the group raised $8,000 for the hospital, equivalent currently to $120,000. In 1919, they raised $9,000.

In preparation for transforming the defunct Maimonides into Mount Sinai, Kurtzon created a reorganization committee. There was an election for regular officers and a board of twenty-one directors. The committee raised $15,000 to cover the remaining money needed to open the hospital. Prominent members of the reorganization committee who played an influential part in the creation of the hospital included J. Bernard, Marcus Bowski, Mrs. Edwin Romburg, Mrs. Ingasy Price, Mr. and Mrs. Meyer Elstein, Mrs. Jacob N. Grosburg, Henry Rieceman, and George Fine. The hospital included many women among its early supporters.

On the brink of realizing his dream, Kurtzon received a letter from the University of Illinois offering to buy the hospital and its grounds for $75,000. He declined the offer, determined to build a hospital for Chicago's Jewish community.

Mount Sinai opened in 1919 with sixty beds, and offered Jewish religious services to patients as well as kosher food. The Eastern European immigrant community in Lawndale organized community bazaars and other events to raise money to help maintain the hospital.

## THE HOSPITAL GROWS

Mount Sinai Hospital began to grow and expand almost immediately. After seven months of operation, doctors at the hospital had treated over one thousand patients and delivered close to two hundred babies.

In 1920, the school of nursing opened.

In 1937, the hospital underwent a major expansion when more floors were added. The hospital would eventually reach eleven floors.

In 1942, hospital fundraisers created the Woman's Board. The board founded thrift shops, in which they sold donated clothing, furniture, and other items to raise money for the hospital. The Woman's Board remains active today, both as a fundraiser and as a goodwill ambassador for the hospital, and has contributed over $3 million to Mount Sinai Hospital.

Shortly after 1945, the Leopold Kling Auditorium was added to the main hospital building, which became a center for teaching, cultural, and social activities. It included a lecture hall, as well as areas for physical training and athletic facilities.

Thirty years after its opening, Mount Sinai had grown considerably. Documents from that period show that in 1949 the hospital admitted ten thousand patients per year and treated over forty-six thousand in the clinics. In 1948, seventeen hundred babies were born at Mount Sinai, one hundred of which were treated in the premature station.

The hospital had 422 beds. At the time, there were eighteen departments, three hundred staff doctors, and twenty-five medical residents and interns on staff. The hospital employed seven hundred employees.

Operating costs were approximately $2 million a year. Paying patients covered $1.6 million, and charitable donations from the Jewish United Fund of Chicago and private donors provided the rest.

## Chapter Two

———

# THE FORMATIVE PERIOD

## HOSPITAL EXPANSIONS IN THE 1950S

In 1958, Mount Sinai opened a major blood bank. It was overseen by Dr. Israel Davidsohn, an internationally acclaimed researcher and chairman of pathology at Mount Sinai, and Dr. Charles Lee.

Under their leadership, the blood center at Mount Sinai developed an outstanding reputation and became the blood center for many other Chicago hospitals. Here, blood was prepared for transfusions. It also became an educational resource, training students how to compare and match blood for transfusions.

In 1958, the Kling Residence Hall was added to the hospital. This was a major housing unit for interns, medical residents, and fellows of the hospital, who could now live where they worked.

## THE LIFE OF A TEACHING HOSPITAL

In 1958, Mount Sinai became the primary teaching affiliate of the Chicago Medical School. This was a significant gain for the hospital. With this partnership, the hospital was now academic, with a full-time teaching staff and a private attending staff who could help teach medical residents and medical students. Many of the attending staff had conducted research and were quite well known. Sinai was now home to medical students, interns, medical residents, and graduate fellows. The affiliation with Chicago Medical School added to Mount Sinai's identity as a research hospital.

## THE NEIGHBORHOOD EVOLVES

While Mount Sinai was growing during those first thirty years, the demographics of Chicago and Lawndale were changing markedly. By the 1950s, much of the ethnic Jewish population in the Lawndale neighborhood had assimilated into the American culture. Over time, the Jewish community on the West Side moved from North Lawndale to other areas of Chicago and its surrounding suburbs. By 1960, the North Lawndale community had become predominantly African American and the immediately neighboring South Lawndale community was in the early stages of transforming to a predominantly Latino neighborhood, primarily with immigrants from Mexico.

## THE FINANCIAL CRISIS OF 1970

The population shift left the hospital with a serious identity crisis. Mount Sinai had been founded with the intention of serving a largely Eastern European Jewish community that was less secure financially than the German Jewish community that had settled on the South Side. While Mount Sinai Hospital continued to serve parts of the Jewish community, including those without insurance, the hospital increasingly primarily served the African American community on the West Side. By 1970, the hospital's payer mix was predominantly dependent on Medicaid, which paid substantially less than commercial insurance, and the percentage of uninsured patients had also risen. The board of the hospital faced a major decision. Should the hospital follow the Jewish community and move to a location where the payer mix would be less challenging or should it stay and serve the North Lawndale community regardless of the financial challenges?

Despite the financial issues, the hospital board decided

it had made a commitment to the Lawndale community. The board of directors decided that they would continue to serve the local community. Their decision was based on the Jewish concept of *tikkun olam*, a Hebrew term that refers to "repair of the world." The Jewish community continued to provide help to support the hospital. The hospital made up the difference by borrowing money and seeking out new sources of revenue. Despite the financial issues, the hospital continued to grow and expand. While this was a difficult period for the hospital financially, it was a successful time in other ways. Mount Sinai had always strived to be close to the Jewish community, and now they had to develop those same close ties with the new residents of the area. Hospital staff attended local churches and community events to help build important bonds. They were on the path to becoming a model of healthcare for underserved communities.

In 1970, a major addition made possible by a philanthropic gift, the Olin-Sang Pavilion, was erected. This pavilion gave the hospital space to accommodate more beds as well as additional laboratory and library space.

In 1976, an oncology unit was opened to simplify the special needs, tests, and treatments required by cancer patients. The addition of the parking garage in 1980 was another important development. A birthing center was opened, providing a specialized maternity unit.

During this period, the board decided to invest in the infrastructure of the community in a joint venture with Ryerson Steel Corporation, which was located next to the hospital. This was an important commitment to Lawndale. The hospital began the first construction in the area for decades, building affordable housing. A further $500,000 was invested by the hospital, beneficiaries, and Ryerson Steel over the next five years for housing rehabilitation.

In 1984, a surgical pavilion was opened, subsidized by Rose and Irving Crown. The pavilion consisted of eleven rooms, including an intensive care unit for high-dependency patients. Patients undergoing high-risk surgeries, such as open-heart surgery, and those with complex or severe health problems, were also cared for in the unit.

In 1990, Mount Sinai Hospital received the designation as a Level I trauma center and was one of the ten original trauma centers designated by the State of Illinois in Chicago. Of the original ten, six dropped out because of the financial challenge of providing trauma care. A trauma center receives patients from the emergency room with serious problems that the emergency room cannot handle. The costs are significant. Trauma centers must maintain twenty-four-hour access to a wide range of medical specialties.

## FORMATION OF THE SINAI HEALTH SYSTEM

In 1984, a major development was the formation of the Sinai Health System. The Sinai Health System contains multiple hospitals and a physicians medical group. The system consists of the following entities, which are briefly described.

## MOUNT SINAI HOSPITAL

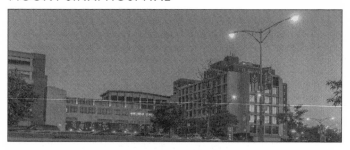

Mount Sinai Hospital is a 432-bed teaching, research, and tertiary care facility. The hospital has two major roles: patient care and community service. Sinai's mission of serving an underserved population was carried out in the hospital.

## HOLY CROSS HOSPITAL

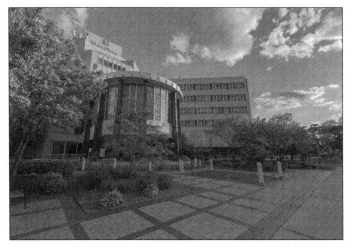

Holy Cross Hospital joined the Sinai Health System in 2013. The hospital was built in Lawndale by the Sisters of Saint Casimir in 1928. At that time, the local population was mainly Lithuanian, Polish, Irish, and German in origin. In the early years, Holy Cross served as the community hospital, receiving fifty thousand emergency visits per year—the largest number in Illinois. During the 1950s, when the demographics of the area began to change, Holy Cross had financial problems and merged with Mount Sinai Hospital. The hospital follows Catholic ethical and religious directives for healthcare.

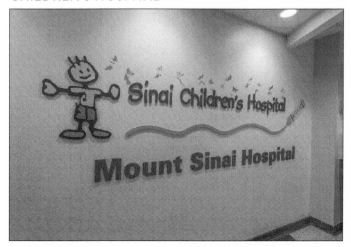

Sinai Children's Hospital was designated as a children's hospital by the State of Illinois in 2004. Sinai Children's Hospital is a "hospital within a hospital" located within Mount Sinai Hospital. Sinai Children's Hospital has provided various levels of pediatric care. As pediatric care has changed, Sinai Children's Hospital has closed its inpatient pediatric services. It continues to provide a high volume of care through its outpatient services and has one of the largest child and adolescent behavioral health programs in Chicago as well. Sinai Children's Hospital also provides a high volume of care through the neonatal intensive care unit and the newborn nursery.

## THE SCHWAB REHABILITATION HOSPITAL

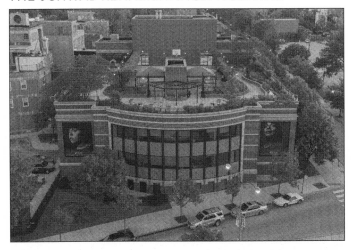

Schwab Rehabilitation Hospital joined the Sinai Health System in 1984. The hospital serves patients with a variety of ailments, including strokes, amputations, spinal cord injury, traumatic brain injury, heart disease, and hepatitis C. Patients are referred to the hospital via other hospitals. In 1998, Schwab opened a new building with additional beds, new therapy units, and a swimming pool for physical therapy. It is one of only two freestanding rehabilitation hospitals in Chicago and the only one in the metropolitan area that primarily treats low-income patients. Patients are referred from hospitals throughout greater Chicago. The training program for medical residents at Schwab is affiliated with the program at the University of Chicago. The program ranks in the nation's top ten resident programs for physical rehabilitation.

## SINAI MEDICAL GROUP

The Sinai Medical Group, which consists of a group of physicians, was created in 2010. The group was formed to fill the vital need for specialty groups in the South and West sides of Chicago. The organization consists of fourteen community-based clinics throughout Chicago. The group employs more than three hundred physicians and over one hundred mid-level providers, covering more than thirty-five specialties. The group treats patients regardless of their ability to pay and works closely with patients to provide affordable healthcare. The group accepts Medicare, Medicaid, and commercial insurance.

SECTION TWO

PROGRESS,
PROGRAMS,
AND PEOPLE

*Chapter Three*

---

# SINAI HEALTH SYSTEM IN THE TWENTIETH AND TWENTY-FIRST CENTURY

During the 1990s, the Sinai Health System launched new initiatives designed to better understand and serve the Lawndale community.

In 1996, with the assistance of funding through the US Department of Housing and Urban Development, Sinai was able to make $100 million in major capital improvements. These included a new emergency room/trauma center, a new obstetrics unit, a new neonatal intensive care unit, and a redesigned front lobby. Sinai has received

$31 million from the City of Chicago TIF (tax increment financing) funding.

In 2009, Mount Sinai received a visit from Vice President Joseph Biden and Secretary of Human Health Services Kathleen Sebelius. They were interested in obtaining insight into how the hospital functioned and seeing how Sinai was coping with and implementing the changes suggested by the Obama administration. The visit was very successful.

In 2015, Sinai developed an association with Ross University Medical School in Barbados. Sinai offers clinical training to students from the medical school.

### SINAI HEALTH SYSTEM TODAY

The hospital's mission has always been to serve its community, and that goal remains the same. In recent years, the hospital has expanded this goal by becoming more involved with community events and organizations, with the aim of further establishing themselves as a trusted community partner.

*Chapter Four*

---

# COMMUNITY PROGRAMS

This chapter describes three major community outreach programs of the Sinai Health System: the Sinai Urban Health Institute (SUHI), the Sinai Community Institute (SCI), and the Sinai Behavioral Healthcare Unit (BHU). These three programs have helped Sinai transcend simple healthcare to create new public health strategies.

## SINAI URBAN HEALTH INSTITUTE (SUHI)

Portions of this information about SUHI were obtained from the classic book by Steven Whitman, Ami M. Shah, and Maureen R. Benjamins, *Urban Health: Combating Disparities with Local Data*, published by Oxford University Press, 2010.

The Sinai Urban Health Institute was founded at Sinai in 2001 by Steven Whitman, PhD. The mission was, "To achieve health equity among communities through excellence and innovation in data-driven research, interventions, evaluation, and collaboration."

The intent of SUHI is not only to document disparities in healthcare but also to develop reliable interventions to reduce those disparities. The plan is to provide adequate healthcare to those in underserved communities. The program is founded on the premise that healthcare is a right, not a privilege. The mission is based on the belief that for a hospital to serve a neighborhood well, it is not only necessary to consider traditional medical care but to also consider the state of health in individuals within the community.

SUHI consists of a group of epidemiologists, researchers, and health educators trained to translate data-based research findings into community-based interventions. Since its founding, SUHI's team has grown from a staff of three to a staff of forty. The institute is very highly regarded nationally, has received numerous awards, and has received significant support from government and foundation funding.

SUHI focuses primarily in two areas. The first is research, which includes health equity and assessment research and community health innovations. The second is consulting, which includes community health worker (CHW) consulting through the Center for CHW Research, Outcomes, and Workforce Development (CROWD) and Evaluation Services providing training and consultation on evaluation and capacity building. Current initiatives include Asthma Care Partners, the Chicago Gun Violence Research Collaborative, Controlling Hyperglycemia among Minority Populations, Helping Her Live (a breast cancer awareness and outreach program), Social Determinants of Health Training for Health Professionals, Evaluation Services, and analysis of racial disparities across the fifty biggest cities in the United States.

## THE SINAI MODEL

Under its founder, Dr. Steve Whitman, SUHI created the Sinai Model to describe an approach to its mission, which is, "To achieve health equity among communities through excellence and innovation in data-driven research, interventions, evaluation, and collaboration." The mission dictates that data are not collected and analyzed purely for scientific advancement; rather, the data are one crucial step in the process of creating change within the communities that are served.

Steps in creating the SUHI model:

1. Collect and analyze data in conjunction with the community, using sound methods.
2. Disseminate the findings. Report back to community members and groups.
3. Develop intervention(s) after the community has identified key problems and possible partners.
4. Obtain funding and implement interventions.
5. Evaluate. Determine effectiveness and sustainability of the SUHI approach.

SUHI has played a major role in conducting community-based research in two of the largest community-driven, face-to-face surveys ever conducted in Chicago. The most recent was Community Health Counts, the Sinai Community Health Survey 2.0, which surveyed over two thousand people in nine Chicago neighborhoods. The information was obtained via door-to-door, face-to-face interviews. Interviewers asked over five hundred questions covering a broad range of topics including physical and mental health, utilization of healthcare resources, and social issues.

The survey showed that major health disparities were observed in all the communities. The disparities included issues such as food insecurity, increased symptoms of post-traumatic stress disorders, lack of health insurance in one in five adults, higher smoking rates, and intimate partner violence in approximately one in three women.

The findings led to three conclusions:

- It is necessary to study these issues on a neighborhood level rather than on a city-wide level.
- There may be alarming health inequalities unobserved in communities.
- To help individuals achieve health equality, it is necessary to understand how social factors may impact community health.

The survey provides the necessary information for the formation of a broad multi-sector partnership between SUHI and the community.

The founder of SUHI, Steve Whitman, PhD, died in 2014. He had received numerous awards and citations and is the basis for SUHI's remarkable development and success. The new president of SUHI, Dr. Sharon Homan, has continued that legacy and substantially expanded SUHI's reach in the community. Under Dr. Homan's leadership SUHI has formed new academic partnerships, grown SUHI's innovative community health worker program and was one of the leaders in establishing the Chicago Gun Violence Research Collaborative which has brought together major academic institutions to provide insights on Chicago's epidemic of gun violence.

## THE SINAI COMMUNITY INSTITUTE (SCI)

Sinai Community Institute was incorporated in 1993 by the Sinai Health System Board of Directors, who were deeply rooted in the Jewish tradition *tikkun olam*...to heal the world. It was the board's core belief that through SCI, a comprehensive array of public health, referral, and social service programs designed to meet the community's most pressing needs would enable the lives of individuals and families served by Sinai Health System to improve.

SCI has established one of the broadest approaches to community interventions of any health system in the United States. Approximately fourteen thousand families each year benefit from SCI's services, from infants to adolescents to adults. This holistic approach has a positive impact on individuals and the community and is part of the belief, similar to SUHI's, that to serve its neighbors well, it must treat the community as well as the hospital inpatients.

Sinai Community Institute's guiding tenets are:

- **Asset focused:** Sinai Community Institute helps clients recognize their strengths and identify their untapped human resources.
- **Partnership:** Sinai Community Institute works in cooperation with Sinai Health System and other community organizations to offer resources that benefit its clients and the community.

- **Solution focused**: Services are created from an understanding of the community environment and designed to address community need.
- **Family-based**: Programs and services focus on families. Intensive case management is a service delivery model by which SCI is able to identify and eliminate barriers that impact the social well-being and health status of individuals, families, and the community.

## HOW SCI PROVIDES SERVICES

SCI uses trained professional and credentialed case managers to provide:

- Comprehensive in-home assessment, which includes:
  - psycho/socio/financial benefit/educational assessment
  - environmental assessment
  - health history
  - risk assessment(s): for example, safety, abuse, mental health, and cognitive difficulties
- Care planning implementation and coordination, which includes:
  - minimum of monthly home visits
  - monitoring establishment of services and referrals
- Case closure, which includes:
  - transition to the highest level of function possible

- ○ attain the best possible outcome
- ○ assure needs have been met

## SCI PROGRAMS, SERVICES, AND RESOURCES
### Support Strong Healthy Families

- Women, Infants, and Children
- Sinai Adult Protective Services
- Family Case Management
- Sinai Better Birth Outcomes
- Health Works of Illinois
- Sinai Senior Centers

### Develop the Potential of Children and Youth

- Early Childhood Development/Prevention Initiative
- Learn Together Afterschool Program
- One Summer Chicago Plus Program
- The Leadership Academy
- Restoring Individuals through Supportive Environments

### Build Strong Community Partnerships

- Sinai Health Ministry Program
- Sinai Community Relations
- Sinai Volunteer and Community Services

Enhance Economic Opportunities

- Workforce Development
- Sinai Technology Center

## SINAI'S BEHAVIORAL HEALTHCARE SERVICES

Sinai Health System has a comprehensive behavioral healthcare program in both its Mount Sinai and Holy Cross campuses. The programs include adult, child, and adolescent behavioral healthcare services. The units manage abnormalities in patient behavior, including mental health issues such as depression. Individuals suffering from behavioral health issues are at increased risk for physical health problems because their condition may cause them to neglect their health. The behavioral health care center provides patients with therapies to help improve their mental health problems.

Sinai's behavioral healthcare program also has a child and adolescent outpatient healthcare program, Under the Rainbow. The children's program is quite popular and offers treatments for an array of pediatric behavioral health issues. The program also has a strong community presence. Clinicians from the program visit schools and provide therapy to individual families. It is a major provider of healthcare for children.

Holy Cross Hospital also has a crisis stabilization unit,

which is the only program of its kind in Chicago. It is a unit in which patients with behavioral health problems can be held for up to thirty-six hours for observation, for assessment of their behavioral health. Patients who do not need hospitalization can then be referred to outpatient services. The unit collaborates with the Chicago Police Department and the Cook County Jail and has been highly successful in reducing emergency room and inpatient utilization.

*Chapter Five*

---

# QUALITY CONTROL
# AND PLANNING

To monitor the success and effectiveness of Sinai's health programs, there are two quality control programs: the Quality and Clinical Integration Unit and the Patient Experience Office, with support from the information services department.

## THE ROLE OF INFORMATION TECHNOLOGY

The information services department at Sinai provides support and resources for hospital-wide data collection. They also provide support to other data collection groups and research groups that are engaged with patients. The unit helps the hospital track and monitor patients and keeps integrated electronic medical records. In addition to this daily support, the group develops algorithms

that can help predict when a patient might require help
or intervention.

## STRATEGIC PLANNING AND MARKETING PROGRAM

The hospital's relatively new Strategic Planning and Marketing Program oversees and coordinates all strategic
planning and implementation of marketing efforts for
the entire Sinai Health System. One of their major proj-
ects has been the implementation of initiatives to build
the hospital's brand. The brand message is: "Be stronger.
Care Harder. Love Deeper." This slogan appears to be
a way of reaching out to people with an engaging and
impactful message that resonates with the community.

# ORGANIZATION

*Chapter Six*

———

# HOSPITAL DEPARTMENTS AND RESEARCH INITIATIVES

This chapter describes the medical departments at Sinai and the research they are performing.

The departments include internal medicine, family medicine, obstetrics/gynecology, pediatrics, radiology, pathology, nuclear medicine, anesthesia, psychiatry, nursing, and pharmacy.

## CURRENT ACTIVE RESEARCH INITIATIVES
### THE CARDIOLOGY DEPARTMENT

The department publishes up to ten original scientific papers every year and has been featured in seventy-four scientific publications. The department's clinical research has led to many awards and honors.

The department was a recipient of a Robert Wood Johnson grant, receiving $269,000 to study and develop solutions to reduce racial and ethnic disparities. This was in collaboration with New York University and George Washington University.

### THE ONCOLOGY DEPARTMENT

The department does clinical cancer research, most notably research on breast cancer. They use clinical trials to evaluate effective cancer treatment approaches. At present, Sinai's oncology department has thirty-seven open clinical trials, in collaboration with Northwestern University and the Eastern Cooperative Group. Members of the department have also published nine papers and nine abstracts detailing and supporting their approach to the treatment of cancer patients. As a result, the department received a Gold Award for participation in research and clinical trials.

## THE HEMATOLOGY DEPARTMENT

The department has published more than 100 research papers. The studies have examined a variety of research studies. They include examination of red blood cells and the bone marrow, studies of lymphocyte properties and their significance, arylesterases and carboxypeptidase values in normal and pathological blood, and genetic studies. The hematologic studies and the genetic study were mainly examined in sickle cell blood and in the bone marrow. Dr Westerman invented the Westerman-Jensen biopsy needle, which allows for simple histologic examination of the bone marrow.

## THE INFECTIOUS DISEASE DEPARTMENT

The unit works with the diagnoses and treatment of communicable diseases. Much of their work is centered around the spread and prevention of HIV and hepatitis C. The department tracks and estimates incidents of HIV infection using a population-based serological method. To date, the unit has published forty-five scientific papers and thirty-five abstracts. They have received multiple grants of up to $1 million to help with the diagnosis and treatment of all infectious diseases in collaboration with the University of Chicago.

## THE RENAL DEPARTMENT

The dialysis program of the renal department is one of the original dialysis units in Chicago. Research activities include development of new dialysis machines and clinical studies of mineral metabolism and anemia in patients with chronic renal disease. The unit also does longitudinal studies on patients with post-infectious glomerulonephritis. Presentations have been made at national meetings.

## THE TRAUMA CENTER

The trauma center is one of the busiest in Illinois. Clinicians in the trauma center have published thirty-one scientific papers and have conducted more than fifty research studies on the positive effects, side effects, dosages, and a comparison of the effects of many drugs.

## THE EMERGENCY DEPARTMENT

The department has received many accolades. A key piece of research is their study of the behavioral aspects of diseases in the emergency room. Papers have been published in eighty-seven scientific journals.

## RESIDENT RESEARCH ACTIVITY

Medical resident research is very active. Research varies

according to the specialty in which the resident is training. The residents present their findings at an annual Resident Day Program. Panels of judges select nine winners, who receive prizes.

## A LEGACY OF RESEARCH

Since Sinai's founding, there has been a considerable amount of internationally acclaimed research at Sinai. From the very beginning, Morris Kurtzon encouraged research as a major goal of the hospital.

### RENOWNED PAST RESEARCHERS

- Dr. Israel Davidsohn was an internationally acclaimed researcher and a pioneering figure in the field of immunohematology. He coauthored more than 150 papers and wrote four books on the subject.
- Dr. Aldo Luisada, cardiology, 1954–1971
- Dr. Chang Lee, blood bank studies, 1957–1983
- Dr. Hyman Zimmerman, hepatology studies, 1946–1963

### EARLY RESEARCHERS (1920–1929)

- Dr. Isadore Trace, studies in cardiology
- Dr. Maurice Tillison, studies on the pathology of obesity

- Dr. Prily Ellis and Dr. Harry Isaac, examiners of electrocardiology
- Dr. Alvin Strauss, innovative work on gastrointestinal surgery
- Dr. Victor Schrager, general surgery
- Dr. Harry Ricktor, thyroid surgery
- Dr. Charles Jacobs, orthopedic surgery

## ALUMNI OF DEPARTMENTAL TRAINING PROGRAMS

- Dr. Gary Maker, professor of surgery at the University of Illinois
- Dr. Harvey Luthra, chief of rheumatology at the Mayo Clinic
- Dr. S.T. Ko, laparoscopic surgery
- Dr. Mohan Airan, laparoscopic procedure for cholecystectomy

*Chapter Seven*

———

# THE ROLE OF PHILANTHROPY IN THE SINAI HEALTH SYSTEM

Philanthropy plays a crucial role in supporting Sinai Health System. Most patients at Sinai are recipients of Medicare or Medicaid or they are uninsured. At the same time, Sinai has a policy of never refusing care to those in need. Sinai often relies on charitable contributions to enhance its vital work. Philanthropic resources at Sinai come in many shapes and forms and they also come from a diverse range of sources. Much of Sinai's philanthropic revenue comes through local and national foundations. Other sources include prominent individuals throughout the Chicago community and corporations that are head-quartered in Chicago.

Sinai is also grateful for its auxiliary boards, Friends of Sinai Children and the Woman's Board. Friends of Sinai Children is comprised of young professionals from Chicago, and they mainly support pediatric programs. The Woman's Board has contributed millions of dollars to Sinai since the 1980s. The Woman's Board is led by a dedicated group of volunteers, who operate the Mount Sinai Hospital Resale Shop on the north side of Chicago. The Resale Shop is a separate 501(c)(3), and with the proceeds from the sales the Woman's Board has contributed millions of dollars to Sinai since the 1980s.

*Chapter Eight*

---

# THE BOARD OF DIRECTORS

The hospital board of directors oversees the hospital system, provides strategic direction, and sets the broad general policies for the hospital. As of October 2018, the current board chair is Robert Markin and the vice chair is Laurie Hernandez.

The board is comprised of twenty-five executives and professionals from Chicago, who are dedicated to donating their time, expertise, and financial resources to Sinai. They also offer connections to corporations, foundations, and other individuals who may be interested in becoming involved at Sinai.

*Chapter Nine*

# THE ADMINISTRATIVE OFFICERS

As of February 2018, the senior administrative officers have included Karen Teitelbaum, president and chief executive officer; Lori Pacura, president of acute care hospitals for Sinai Health System; Jason N. Spigner, chief human resources officer; Roberta Rakove, senior vice president of external affairs and strategy for Sinai Health System; Dr. Sharon Homan, president of the Sinai Urban Institute; Debra Wesley, president of Sinai Community Institute; Ed Carne, president of Sinai Medical Group; Dr. Michelle Gittler, medical director of Schwab Rehabilitation Hospital; Dr. Maria Iliescu-Levine, chief medical officer of Sinai Health; and Airica Steed, Chief Operating Officer for Sinai Health System.

*Chapter Ten*

---

# AWARDS AND RECOGNITION

The hospital and staff have received an array of awards over the decades for clinical excellence and advancements in medical research. This is an extensive but not exhaustive list of notable or significant accolades the Sinai Health System and its illustrious staff have been awarded.

## SIGNIFICANT AWARDS

- Illinois Hospital Association Quality Award
- First Quality Award, 2015—presented to Sinai Health System for the paper, "Helping Adults Breathe and Thrive: A Healthy Home Approach to Improving Respiratory Health of Adults with Asthma"
- Pledge Quality Achievement Award
- Foster McGraw Award, 1992—given to the hospital

in recognition of the outstanding service it provides to the community

- Robert Wood Johnson Award—recognizes individuals who have successfully implemented effective system changes. Awarded to the hospital in 2007 for fighting childhood obesity and again in 2016 for health equity.
- Stroke Gold Plus Quality Achievement Award, 2015—Awarded by the American Heart Association/ American Stroke Association. This awarding body recognizes hospitals that ensure stroke patients receive the most appropriate treatment according to national guidelines.
- Illinois Council of Health-System Pharmacists (ICHP) Best Practice Award, 2015—for the Better Bones for Babies Program
- Mount Sinai's Cancer program was awarded a certificate of excellence by the American Society of Clinical Oncology.
- Deaf Illinois award for Best Health Services, 2007, 2009, and 2011
- The Organ and Tissue Network Gift of Hope, Silver Medal of Honor—Sinai is named a lifesaving partner for support of organ and tissue donations.
- Nurse Executive of the Year Award, 2017—awarded to Mary Gollinger, the vice president of Schwab Rehabilitation Hospital
- Two prestigious Quality of Care Awards from the Quality Institute of Illinois and the Bosco Association

# CONCLUSION

The story of the Sinai Health System is the story of a pioneering hospital system that has successfully helped integrate roughly 200,000 Jewish refugees into the United States. Although significant changing demographics occurred in the community, the hospital continued to provide quality care to the community. The hospital has had a rich research background since its founding.

The Sinai Model, founded at Sinai, has been accepted nationally as a successful model for providing healthcare for underserved communities.

# ACKNOWLEDGMENTS

First, I would like to thank the many interviewees, approximately two hundred, who provided a considerable amount of information about Sinai and in many ways introduced me to the hospital.

I very much appreciate the very high level of support given by Professor Robert Souhami and Allan Morales.

I further appreciate the critical reviews by Jade Dell, Rabbi Howard Berman, Dr. Stuart Kiken, Jeff Westerman, and Mark Westerman.

I would further like to thank Karen Teitelbaum, president of the Chicago Sinai Health System, who has made this book possible.

The support given by former presidents of Sinai Alan Channing, Benn Greenspan, and Ruth Rothstein has been considerable.

Many thanks to Roberta Rakove and Dianne Hunter for administrative support.

# ABOUT THE AUTHOR

MAXWELL P. WESTERMAN, MD, has been practicing medicine for over 65 years. During that time, he has been a physician, educator and researcher. Dr. Westerman has published numerous basic research articles on patients with sickle cell disease, and in 1958 invented the first bone marrow biopsy needle—the Westerman-Jensen biopsy needle—which was the first simple method for obtaining bone marrow tissue for diagnosis and study of marrow. He first began working at Mount Sinai in 1968 as a senior attending physician and chief of hematology and oncology. He has taught medicine at the University of Pittsburgh Medical School, Chicago Medical School, and Rush Medical College.

Made in the USA
Columbia, SC
07 June 2019